THE COVID "VACCINE", A DANGER TO THE SOUL?

a Christian perspective

Orsolya Eden

Imprint:

*Orsolya Eden**
c/o AutorenServices.de
Birkenallee 24
36037 Fulda
Germany

* Please don´t send any parcels to this address. If you would like to send a parcel to me, please enquire

first via e - mail for a separate address.
Thank you for your understanding.

E - mail:
Orsolyaeden1@use.startmail.com

Cover design, illustration and photos: Orsolya Eden
Translation from German into English: Orsolya Eden
Note: Orsolya Eden is a pen name.
ISBN paperback:
978-3-949222-43-6

Notice:

The information in this booklet is without warranty; it is merely the personal opinion of the author.

It is not a medical recommendation.

Glory be to the Father and the Son and the Holy Spirit and gratitude be to the Blessed Virgin Mary and to St. Joseph

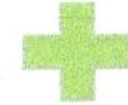

"I am the way, the truth and the life. No one comes to the Father except through me."

Jesus Christ
(John, 14, 6-7)

The Covid "Vaccine" - a curse or a blessing?

It does not matter who the manufacturer of the vaccine is, because in the end, all "vaccines" are not "vaccines" in the conventional sense, but constitute a gene therapy. Everyone is free to have his or her opinion about vaccination in the "true" meaning of the word, but what disconcerts me particularly with the Covid-Vaccine is, that each person who is "vaccinated" regains his/her civil rights, because he/she is supposedly no longer contagious.[1] That is, the “vaccinated” person gets his "old" life back, so to speak. And what will become of the others? What will happen to those who do not want to get "vaccinated" for health reasons, or who have ethical and other concerns? Will they still be allowed to

---

[1] Recent studies suggest that the „vaccine“ only allows for a milder course.

travel, attend school or even go to work?

If you look towards Israel, the "non-vaccinated" are excluded from economic and social life.

At first they are suspended from their jobs and then dismissed. So, even though perhaps no one is directly forced to be "vaccinated", there is an indirect compulsion to get “vaccinated”. After all, who can afford to give up his/her job or to dispense of the education for the children?

This compulsion reminds me strongly of the Book of Revelation in the New Testament of the Bible. In Rev 13:12-18 the following is stated:

"12 And all the power of the first beast it exercises before it, and it causes the earth and those who dwell on it to worship the first beast, whose death wound has been healed. 13 And he does great signs, that he himself causes fire to come down from heaven to the earth before men; 14 And he deceives those who dwell on the earth because of the signs which it was given him to do before the beast, and he tells those who dwell on the earth to make an image to the beast who has the wound of the sword and ⟨has come to life again⟩. 15 And it was given to him to give breath to the image of the beast,[2] so that the image of

---

[2] Just a thought: Could this section refer to humanoid robots, like Sophia made by

the beast even spoke and caused all to be killed who did not worship the image of the beast. 16 **And it causeth all, both small and great, and rich and poor, and free and bond, to receive a mark in their right hand, or in their foreheads; 17 and that no man might buy or sell, save he that receiveth the mark, the name of the beast or the number of its name. 18 Here is wisdom. He who has**

Hanson Robotics (i.e. artificial intelligence)?

understanding, calculate the number of the beast! For it is the number of a man; and his number is 666.
Now it must be known that anyone who accepts the mark of the beast is excluded from the glory of God, i.e., he is punished by death in the lake of fire (Rev 19:20).
On the other hand, whoever does not accept the mark will reign with Christ for 1000 years. (Rev 20,4)
Even if the "vaccination" is not yet administered on the

palm of the hand or on the forehead, the administration of the vaccine acts in some countries, and may eventually act in all parts of the world, like the mark of the beast. For without a Covid - 19 vaccination card, many, if not all civil rights are/will be taken away.
The vaccination passport/card will soon be redundant, if that´s not already the case. As several doctors, like Dr. Carrie Madej

state that[3], e.g., in the Moderna Vaccine, the oxidative enzyme Luciferase (derived from Lucifer, the light bearer) is already contained.

Luciferase is already widely used in cancer research. The

---

[3] Dr Carrie Madej has an urgent warning about the upcoming covid -19 vaccines, under: https://www.bitchute.com/video/z9T8D754Uews/ (retrieved on 12 April 2021).

Dr. Carrie Madej - Medical Professionals That Speak Out under: https://www.bitchute.com/video/dkz7pPRNSbJ8/ (retrieved on 12 April 2021).

Hydrogel microbots to ferry living cells under: https://www.youtube.com/watch?v=mmC2cJeK6nk (retrieved on 12 April 2021).

Enzyme is invisible from the outside, but detectable by use of a scanner.
Also, the application of the “vaccine“ could be simplified. The reknowned Massachusetts Institute of Technology (MIT) introduces the so-called “quantum dot tattoo“ vaccination plaster. It consists of 100 microneedles which contain the serum. Once applied, these needles dissolve underneath the skin. Hence the plaster can be easily applied on the hand and is

almost painless. Thus, the inclusion of Luciferase into the vaccine enables self-vaccination, since the status of vaccination is scannable.[4] I cannot say whether there are actually nanosensors embedded in a hydrogel in the "vaccines" which in turn connect you to the internet and facilitate the sending and

---

[4] Anne Trafton, Massachusetts Institute of Technology, *MIT NEWS Storing medical information below the skin's surface*, 18 December 2019, under: https://news.mit.edu/2019/storing-vaccine-history-skin-1218 (retrieved on 3 May 2021).

receiving of information. But if you read the package inserts of the "vaccine" manufacturers, they do talk about nanoparticles embedded in lipids. What kind of particles are involved is not explained any further. It is important to know that this technology already exists. The company Profusa, for example, presents this technology on its website.[5]

---

[5] Profusa Inc. under: https://profusa.com/video/ und https://profusa.com/injectable-body-sensors-take-personal-chemistry-to-a-cell-phone-closer-to-reality/ (retrieved on 9 June 2021).

Also, in 2018, Microsoft applied for a patent on how to connect humans to the digital payment system (cryptocurrency).[6] That the "vaccines" are gene therapy and not classical vaccinations is clear from the "instruction leaflets", which, by the way, are accessible to everyone at least online. So, after this

---

[6] Espacenet Patent search, CRYPTOCURRENCY SYSTEM USING BODY ACTIVITY DATA WO2020060606A1 • 2020-03-26 • MICROSOFT TECHNOLOGY LICENSING LLC [US] Earliest priority: 2018-09-21 under: https://worldwide.espacenet.com/patent/search/family/067396975/publication/WO2020060606A1?q=microsoft%20cryptocurrency (retrieved on 15 May 2021).

gene therapy, we could be like genetically manipulated plants. This is an active intervention in God's creation and we are not told what the consequences for us will be. It is also of considerable importance that the RNA used by the pharmaceutical industry is synthetic and therefore patentable. Hence, part of my DNA could belong to a company in the future!!! Outrageous, yes. This context is intertwined with other topics, such as "transhumanism" and "neurolink". (the fusion of man and machine) As far as faith is concerned, the whistleblower Joey Lambardi goes as far as to claim that one can already (via fun vax) do away with faith by way of vaccination. If one is reluctant to believe in the existence of the nanosensors, despite of all the evidence, according to Dr. Tenpenny, the "vaccination" will definitely have negative effects on our autoimmune system, which in some cases can (drastically) shorten our

lives.[7] The question also needs to be raised if the “vaccinated“, due to a weakened immune system, are more susceptible to new viral diseases than “unvaccinated “people.
I think that if there is only a grain of truth in these statements, it is worth pursuing them, because this

---

[7] ALEX JONES (2nd HOUR) Friday 3/5/21 • DR. SHERRI TENPENNY, News, Reports & Analysis • Infowars under: https://www.bitchute.com/video/0ezmweGU65TJ/ (retrieved on 13 April 2021).

technology threatens us as a species.
Once the Covid-19 "vaccine" is applied as a quantum dot tattoo[8] and linked to the planned digital identification number worn on the body

---

[8] Anne Trafton, Massachusetts Institute of Technology, *MIT NEWS Storing medical information below the skin's surface*, 18 Dezember 2019, under: https://news.mit.edu/2019/storing-vaccine-history-skin-1218 (retrieved on 3. May 2021).

(ID2020),[9] for me at least, the criteria of the mark of the beast according to the Revelation of John, are definitively fulfilled. Some sources claim, that the Federal Government of Germany, e.g., has already passed the law for the implementation of ID 2020.[10]

---

[9] *eClinic Learning in OFF GRID HEALTHCARE, ID2020 Alliance: Global Mandatory Vaccinations + Biometric ID Integration*, 20 Dezember 2019, under: https://eclinik.net/id2020-alliance-global-mandatory-vaccinations-biometric-id-integration/ (retrieved on 3 May 2021).

[10] Norbert Haering, Geld und mehr under: https://norberthaering.de/die-regenten-der-

It is well known, that corona viruses have been around for a long time, and that this new strain of the virus only appeared in 2019, hence the abbreviation Covid - 19. Even if this new strain really exists, a question arises. How could a Richard Rothchild from London have already applied for a patent in 2015, for a testing procedure of Covid - 19?[11] Alternative media often

---

welt/bundestag-buergernummer/, (retrieved on 10 May 2021).

[11] Espcaenet Patent Search, US2020279585A1 System and Method for

talks of Hydroxychloroquine and Ivermectin[12] as a remedy, as well as a preventative for Corona. Suramin, a drug produced by the pharmaceutical company Bayer, is also being traded as an "antidote" for the artificial spike proteins that are in the

---

Testing for COVID-19, Rothschild, Richard A., Priority Date: US201562240783P·2015-10-13; under: https://worldwide.espacenet.com/patent/search/family/072235969/publication/US2020279585A1?q=rothschild%20covid%2019 (retrieved on 10 May 2021).

[12]CANST under: https://www.bitchute.com/video/4TcyukoPo0uq/ (retrieved on 10 May 2021).

body after “vaccination” or as a preventative against shedding from “vaccinated” people.[13] [14] Furthermore, shikimic acid (contained in fennel and star anise), nano soma, and the drug

---

[13] Hugo4NWQ under: https://www.bitchute.com/video/VRmWEgLb9j0Z/ (retrieved on June 18 2021).

[14] **Advisory: Dr. Mikovits has distanced herself from the fact that suramin should be contained in pine needles. It is also generally advised to be careful with pine needle tea, as turpentine can be released from the needles when the tea is overheated. Therefore, as a rule of thumb, one should never boil pine needle tea and rather put a silver spoon in the cup.**

Ivermectin are said to have a spike protein destructive effect.[15] [16]

For pregnant women and lactating women, the administration of Suramin, Ivermectin and the Shikimic

---

[15] Spacetravelinalabamacom under: https://spacetravelinalabama.com/2021/05/19/ivermectin-medicine-to-kill-parasites-can-also-kill-darpa-hydrogel-with-nano-parasites/ (retrieved on 18 June 2021).

[16] Survive the News, *Antidote for Spike Proteins & COVID-19 Vaccination? Fennel, Star Anise, Shikimic acid, Pine Tree Needle Turpentine & NANO SOMA,* under: https://www.survivethenews.com/antidote-spike-proteins-covid19-vaccination-fennel-star-anise-pine-needle-tea-turpentine-nano-soma/, (retrieved on 25 June 2021).

acid is not recommended.[17] Everyone, especially pregnant and lactating women, should always seek medical advice before taking any new "medication". Regular administration of vitamin D, vitamin C and zinc is also said to be helpful in shielding against Covid-19.

---

[17] Jacqueline in Deep Roots at Home, *3 Foods That Contain Shikimic Acid to Halt Spike Protein Transmission* under: https://deeprootsathome.com/3-foods-that-contain-shikimic-acid-to-halt-transmission/, retrieved on 25 June 2021).

I have no opinion on these substances, nor do I make any recommendations. This is because I do not want to be guilty in any way. Likewise, I have no opinion on whether the "vaccination" will lead to a Covid - 19 pandemic, since the protein is now in the body, and whether the synthetic spike proteins will be transmitted to the “unvaccinated”. But since real vaccines cause mini-infections, it is only likely

and logical that it is the same with the Covid shot.

We are the living temple of God through our baptism.[18] If we allow our body to be changed by this technique, HE has no place in us anymore.
Too far-fetched? Perhaps that is exactly what 2 Thess 3

---

[18] 1 Cor 3:16 17: "3 Do you not know that you are God's temple and that the Spirit of God dwells in you? 17 If anyone corrupts the temple of God, God will corrupt him; for the temple of God is holy, and that is *you*."

- 5 alludes to. The following is said there: "3 Let no one deceive you! (for that day will not come) unless the apostasy has come first and **the man of lawlessness** has been revealed, the son of perdition, 4 who rebels and exalts himself above all that is called God or is the object of worship, so that he **sits in the temple and pretends to be God**." Could the artificial RNA strand behave as if the Antichrist were sitting on the throne?

If so, then we are understandably excluded from the glory of God according to Rev. 19:20. Is this what we want, to be a human slave machine? Whom then do we serve? Finally, the good news: according to Rev 13:5 and Dan 12:7, the **great** tribulation is supposed to last "only" for about 3.5 years. Even if there is nothing to these statements, I do not want to build my supposed happiness on the misfortune of others. The others, are the aborted fetuses. Without their aid, virtually none of these "vaccines" can be manufactured. Their cells are either contained in the "vaccines" themselves or the active ingredients were tested on these cells in the laboratory.[19] (The chart proving this, as sated by the Charlotte Lozier Institute is reproduced at the end of the book) Also, there seems to be some doubt as to whether

[19] https://s27589.pcdn.co/wp-content/uploads/2020/12/06.02.21-warp-speed-vaccines-June.pdf (retrieved on 15 December 2021).

these fetal cells are really from babies who died by abortion, or whether the babies were still alive after the abortion when the cells were harvested from them.[20] The others are also people, who have sustained health injuries from the "Covid vaccine" and are not even entitled to any compensation. What about

---

[20] LIFE SITE under: https://www.lifesitenews.com/blogs/the-unborn-babies-used-for-vaccine-development-were-alive-at-tissue-extraction (retrieved on 18 June 2021).

the dead we have to mourn as a result of the "vaccines". Are these people just collateral damage. In the USA, all vaccine related deaths are recorded in the database VAERS (Vaccine Adverse Event Reporting System). At this point, almost 6000 people have already died as a result of a Covid 19 "vaccination".[21] Also, about

[21] https://vaers.hhs.gov/index.html (retrieved on 25 June 2021) and Robert F. Kennedy Jr., in Z3News, *Latest VAERS Data Show: 5,165 Deaths Reported Following COVID Vaccines,* under: https://z3news.com/w/latest-vaers-data-show-5165-deaths-reported-following-covid-

250,000 "vaccine victims" have spoken out in the US. In the spirit of "cancel culture", however, Facebook has deleted the post.[22] Recently, the RNA vaccine inventor Dr. Robert Malone has also warned against his own invention. He stated that it among other things can cause myocarditis, as well as

---

vaccines/, 4 June 2021 (retrieved on 25 June 2021.

[22] The Highwire with Del Bigtree, *MRNA VACCINE INVENTOR CALLS FOR STOP OF COVID VAX*, 25. Juni 2021 under: https://www.bitchute.com/video/yn3u9ETcxCbV/, at 1 hr 9 min (retrieved on 27 June 2021).

blood clots and has a negative effect on the reproductive system.[23] These "vaccines" are not licensed (according to the package insert), they only have emergency authorisation, and there are no long-term studies. What if this experiment backfires and after 2 (or more) years many of the “vaccinated” suddenly

[23] The Highwire with Del Bigtree, *MRNA VACCINE INVENTOR CALLS FOR STOP OF COVID VAX*, 25 June 2021 under: https://www.bitchute.com/video/yn3u9ETcxCbV/ (retrieved on 27. June 2021).

die or become severely ill? Why after such a long period of time? Some doctors, like Dr. Tenpenny, assume that the full extent of the shot will only be apparent after such a long period of time.[24] Despite all the drama, let us remember that our Lord has the last word in everything

---

[24] Robert David Steele UNRIG, *Mirror: Dr. Sherri Tenpenny - 8 Ways mRNA COVID Vaccine Can Kill You*, 22. April 2021 under: https://www.bitchute.com/video/JmNwCp5ljt0g/ (retrieved on 27 June 2021).

and can also raise the dead back to life.
Another **comfort** for believers who share my view and must watch how family members being "vaccinated", can be the **Devotion of the "seven Our Fathers and seven Hail Marys in honour of the Precious Blood of Jesus Christ"**. For our Lord promised to the prayerful, through St. Bridget of Sweden, among other things, the following assurances:

"The souls of their relatives unto the fourth generation shall escape hell."[25] (The devotion can be found at the end of this book)

There is also **hope** for those who regret their "vaccination". They always have the possibility of **confession**.
If confession is not available to them, they can in any case pray the **Divine Mercy Chaplet**.

---

[25] Brigitta Prayers, Mediatrix – Verlag D-84503 Altötting, pp. 11, 12.

For Jesus has promised to everyone, that if they prayed this chaplet only once, their soul would no longer perish.[26] Also, the souls for whom one has prayed this chaplet for, especially at the hour of death, are no longer lost.[27]

Of particular value would be the celebration of **Divine**

---

[26] Diary of Sister Faustyna Kowalska 476 du 950), quoted from: Fr. Seraphim Michalenko, MIC together with Vinny Flynn and Robert A. Stackpole, *The Divine Mercy Message and Devotion,* revised edition, MARIAN PRESS, Stockbridge MA 01263, 2008, pp. 65 – 67.

[27] Ibid., p. 548 (1541).

Mercy Sunday on the first Sunday after Easter.
As Our Lord promised to St. Sister Faustina, that whoever goes to Holy Confession and receives Holy Communion on that day will receive forgiveness of all sins and the remission of all penalties.[28] Even the veneration of the image of the Merciful Jesus would already save the soul.[29] (You will find the

[28] Ibid., p. 139 (299 – 300).

[29] Ibid., p. 24 (48).

chaplet and the image at the end of the book)

For the doubters, a few statements straight from the "horse's mouth".

Jacques Attali (former advisor to France's Prime Minister Mitterand[30] made the following statement in an interview: "In the future, it is going to be a case of finding a way to reduce the population. We will start with the "old", because once

---

[30] News! Under:https://www.youtube.com/results?search_query=jacques+attali+%C3%BCber+die+Zukunft+1981 (retrieved on 19 June 2021).

people are over 60, 65, they live longer than they are productive, and that costs society dearly. Then the weak and then the useless who contribute nothing to society because they are becoming an ever increasing number and finally, above all, the stupid. Euthanasia is aimed at these groups. Euthanasia must be an essential tool of our future societies, in all cases. Of course, we will not be able to execute people or organise camps. We will get rid of them by making them believe that it is for their own good. A population that is too large and largely unnecessary is something that is too costly economically. Socially, too, it is much better for the human machine to stop abruptly than to decay gradually. As you can imagine, we will not be able to pass intelligence tests on millions and millions of people. We will find or cause something, a pandemic that will target certain people, a real economic crisis or not, a virus that will affect the old or the elderly. It does not matter. The weak and the fearful will succumb, the stupid will believe and ask to be treated. We will have made sure to have planned the treatment, a treatment that will be the solution. So the selection of the idiots, will take care of itself. They will go to the slaughter by themselves.“

If this is too extreme for you, just look at the World Economic Forum's plans for the global future. Its founder,

Klaus Schwab, publicly advocates for a completely digitised society controlled by AI (artificial intelligence). Ultimately, humans will merge with artificial intelligence, by way of a microchip implant. Schwab calls this the fourth industrial revolution. At the same time, he stresses that the Corona pandemic is a great opportunity for the fourth industrial revolution.[31]

---

[31] Lee Kuan Yew School of Public Policy (LKY School)

24.6K subscribers under: https://www.youtube.com/watch?v=7xUk1F7dyvl (retrieved on 19 June 2021).

Gavi, the Vaccine Alliance, *Gavi@20 - Klaus Schwab (version française)* under: https://www.youtube.com/watch?v=CqtMcdWTUZo (retrieved on 19 June 2021).

World Economic Forum, *When Humans Become Cyborgs | DAVOS 2020*

under: https://www.youtube.com/watch?v=zrNaaz1isEQ (retrieved on 19 June 2021).

The World Knowledge Forum, *COVID-19 and the 4th Industrial Revolution | Klaus Schwab | WKF 2020* under: https://www.youtube.com/watch?v=TZyzI7ojsho (retrieved on 19 June 2021).

Keeping the WEF's goals in mind, perhaps the global vaccination campaigns launched by GAVI (which in turn was created by the WEF) take on a new meaning? It is also rumoured that the PCR tests act like “mini-

---

s0p0a0c0e0, *Klaus Schwab, Fusion du monde physique, digital et biologique (RTS, 10 janvier 2016)* under: https://www.youtube.com/watch?v=uf-l9Sp1nHc (retrieved on 19 June 2021).

vaccinations".[32] Also, many self-test swabs are contaminated by toxic ethylene oxide.[33] Why do we go along with this worldwide? Do allow our children to be re-educated

---

[32] Der Freie, *Achtung wichtig! Ist der PCR-Test die Impfung?*, 12. Oktober 2020 under: https://www.bitchute.com/video/MwmaJ1F4bZsW/ (retrieved on 27 June 2021).

[33] Heike Beier, in Ökotest.de, *Corona-Teststäbchen: Enthalten sie einen krebserregenden Stoff?* under: https://www.oekotest.de/gesundheit-medikamente/Corona-Teststaebchen-Enthalten-sie-einen-krebserregenden-Stoff_11869_1.html, 11. Mai 2021 (retrieved on 27 June 2021).

through regular self-testing in schools, to become neurotics, and to suffer brain damage (through lack of oxygen) by wearing masks all the time? What would Jesus have say to that?

Last but not least, one should know that Pope Francis (knowingly or not) is at the very top of the new global world order. In December 2020, the Vatican joined a coalition for "inclusive capitalism".[34] Furthermore, Pope Francis has spoken out in favour of the Covid injection, as an act

---

[34] Dr Taylor Marshall, *586: Pope Francis & Rothschild partner with "Guardian" CEOs for Vatican Inclusive Capitalism Council [Podcast]* under: https://taylormarshall.com/2020/12/586-pope-francis-rothschild-partner-guardian-ceos-vatican-inclusive-capitalism-council-podcast.html (retrieved on 19 June 2021).

of charity. [35] and let himself be “vaccinated”. Yes, as a believer we have to listen to the Pope in matters of faith. But we must not follow him into sin.[36] [37] Pope Honorious

---

[35] Extrem News, *Impfstoffe und Forschung mit abgetriebenen Fötuszellen: Eine Erinnerung an den neuesten wissenschaftlichen „Durchbruch“*, 21 May 2021 under: https://www.extremnews.com/berichte/gesundheit/be851829fef26eb (retrieved on 25 June 2021).

[36] Father Nicholas Gruner, *CRUCIAL TRUTHS TO SAVE YOUR SOUL*, Immaculate Heart Publications, Buffalo, New York 2014, p. 55.

[37] **Mt 18, 15 - 18: "15 But if your brother sins, go and confront him between you and him**

(approx. 500 – 600 AD), for example, was post hum excommunicated, for having advocated for a false

---

alone. If he listens to you, you have won your brother. 16 But if he does not listen, take one or two more with you, so that from the mouths of two or three witnesses everything may be confirmed. 17 But if he will not hearken unto them, tell it the church, but if he will not hearken also onto the church, let him be unto thee as the Gentile and the tax collector!"

dogma.[38] Cells, of aborted fetuses are included in many vaccines. They are also included in many of the Covid "vaccines." Abortion violates (unless the mother's life is in danger) the 6th commandment ("Thou shalt not kill").[39]

Nearly every year, abortion is the No. 1 cause of death worldwide. In 2019 alone, 42.4 million babies were

---

[38] Father Nicholas Gruner, *CRUCIAL TRUTHS TO SAVE YOUR SOUL*, Immaculate Heart Publications, Buffalo, New York, 2014, p. 132.

[39] Ex 20:13.

aborted (the number of unreported cases is likely much higher).[40] Therefore, significantly more people die from an abortion than due to Covid 19. Aborted people die because they are definitely unwanted. Who has the right to say which human being may live and which one may not. Why are there no measures taken in this case,

---

[40] amazing discoveries, *Sexualerziehung für mehr Abtreibungen*, under: https://www.amazing-discoveries.org/news/sexualerziehung-fuer-mehr-abtreibungen.html (retrieved on 19 June 2021).

to save the lives of these people. Moreover, these are people who are not even able to defend themselves. What kind of a society are we if we murder our own children in order to preserve our own lives?

Our **Lady of Fatima** (approved Marian apparition, Portugal, 1917) pointed out to us that **the means of salvation for our time are the Rosary, the Devotion of**

the 5 First Saturdays[41] and the Consecration of Russia to her Immaculate Heart.
The Consecration of Russia was carried out several times by the Pope, but never completely, because every

---

[41] **The Devotion of the First 5 Saturdays consists of 5 consecutive First Saturdays of the month.
On each Saturday one is asked to pray the holy Rosary, meditate on the mysteries on the Rosary for 15 minutes, go to confession and then to receive the Holy Eucharist with the intention of apologizing for the insults against Our Lady´s Immaculate Heart.**

bishop has to join into the Consecration.

On 25 March 2022, Pope Francis also consecrated Russia to the Immaculate Heart of Our Lady. He invited all bishops to join in the act of Consecration. It is to be hoped that all bishops have heeded his invitation.[42]

---

[42] Armin Berger, BISTUM PASSAU, *Weihe Russlands und der Ukraine an das Herz Mariens, 23.03.2022* under: https://www.bistum-passau.de/artikel/weiheakt-zum-unbefleckten-herzen-mariens (retrieved on 6 May 2022).

Our Lady of La Salette

(approved Marian apparition site, France, 1846)

"If my people will not submit, I am forced to let down the arm of my Son."

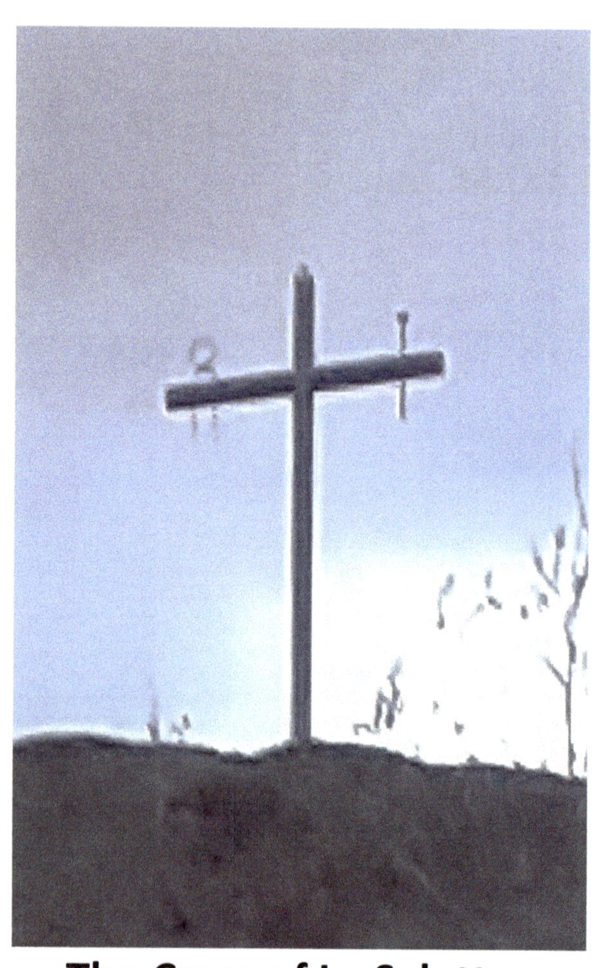

The Cross of La Salette

In **Garabandal** (Marian apparition site in Spain, 1961-65), the last message of the Mother of God was the following:

"Since my message from 18 October 1961 was not heeded and was not made known, I inform you that this is the last message. Beforehand, the chalice was filling up, now it is overflowing. Many cardinals, many bishops and many priests are on the way to perdition, taking many souls

with them. Less and less importance is given to the Eucharist. You should turn the wrath of God away from you through your efforts. If you ask Him for forgiveness with a sincere heart, He will forgive you. I, your Mother, ask you through the intercession of St. Michael the Archangel to change your lives. You are now receiving the final warnings. I love you very much and do not want your damnation. Pray to us sincerely and we will fulfill your requests. You

should make more sacrifices.
Recall the Passion of Jesus."

Apostel Paul
(Ro: 1-2)

"11 Put on the whole armour
of God, that you may be able
to stand against the
cunnings of the devil! 12 For
our struggle is not against
flesh and blood, but against
the powers, against the
authorities, against the
world rulers of this darkness,
against the spiritual

(powers) of wickedness in the heavenly realm."

I wish us all faith in God.

The 7 Our Fathers and 7 Hail Marys (according to the revelation of St. Bridget of Sweden).[43]

"The Divine Saviour revealed to St. Bridget the following promise:

---

[43] This devotion has been approved and recommended by the Sacred Congregation, the Sacro Collegio de propaganda fide, and also by Pope Clement XII (pontificate of 1730-1740). From: "Through Mary to Jesus" p. 186 ff; Mediatrix Publishers.

Know that I will grant 5 graces to those who pray the Seven Our Fathers and Hail Marys in honour of My Precious Blood for 12 years:

1. They will not go to purgatory.

2. I will be included in the number of martyrs, as if they had shed their blood for the faith.

3) I will keep three souls of their relatives in sanctifying grace according to their choice.

4. The souls of their relatives up to the 4th generation will escape hell.

5. They will be notified one month before they die of their imminent death. If they die before that time, I consider it as having been accomplished, that is, as if they had fulfilled this condition.

Pope Innocent X confirmed this revelation and added that the souls who fulfill the revelation will liberate one soul from Purgatory every Good Friday. This devotion can easily be combined with the veneration and sacrifice of the Holy Wounds of our Saviour, as the Precious Blood flowed from His wounds. The Saviour recommended this exercise to Sister Mary Martha Chambon and in exchange gave her great promises. It is recommended to add the following prayers to the 7 Our Fathers:

Before the beginning:

"O Jesus, I will now pray the Our Father seven times, in union with the love in which Thou hast sanctified and sweetened this prayer in Thy heart. Receive it from my lips into Thy Divine Heart, improve and perfect it so much that it may give as much honour and joy to the Most Holy Trinity as Thou didst give it on earth with this prayer, and may these overflow to Thy most holy humanity for the glorification of Thy holy wounds and of the Precious Blood which Thou didst shed from them."

1. The circumcision:

"Our Father...

Eternal Father, through the Immaculate Hands of Mary and the Divine Heart of Jesus, I offer You the first wounds, the first pains, and the first shedding of Blood of Jesus for the expiation of my and all men's sins of youth and for the prevention of first mortal sins, especially in my kinship.

Hail Mary...

2. The sweating of blood:

"Our Father...

Eternal Father, through the Immaculate Hands of Mary and the Divine Heart of Jesus, I offer you the terrible sufferings of the Heart of Jesus on Mount of Olives and every drop of His bloody sweat for the expiation of my sins of the heart and those of all men, for the prevention of such sins and for the increase of the love for God and for the love of neighbour.

Hail Mary..."

3. The flagellation:

"Our Father...

Eternal Father, through the Immaculate Hands of Mary and the Divine Heart of Jesus, I offer you the thousands of wounds, the cruel pains and the Precious Blood of Jesus of the flagellation for the expiation of my and all men's sins of the flesh, for the prevention of such sins and for the preservation of the innocence, especially in my kinship.

Hail Mary ..."

4. The crowning with thorns:

"Our Father ...

Eternal Father, through the Immaculate Hands of Mary

and the Divine Heart of Jesus, I offer You the wounds, pains, and Precious Blood of the Holy Head of Jesus from the Crowning with Thorns in reparation for my sins of the Spirit and those of all men, for the prevention of such sins, and for the spread of the Kingship of Christ on earth.

Hail Mary...

5. The carrying of the cross:

"Our Father...

Eternal Father, through the Immaculate Hands of Mary and the divine Heart of Jesus, I offer You the sufferings of Jesus on His Way of the Cross, especially of His sacred shoulder wound and its precious blood in reparation for my and all men's rebellion against the Cross and murmuring against Your holy orders and all other sins of the tongue, for the prevention of such sins and for true love of the Cross.

Hail Mary..."

6. The crucifixion of Jesus:

"Our Father...

Eternal Father, through the Immaculate Hands of Mary and the Divine Heart of Jesus, I offer You Your Son on the cross, His nailing and exaltation, His wounds on hands and feet and the three streams of His Holy Blood that gushed from them, His extreme poverty, all His bodily and mental agonies, His precious death and its bloodless renewal in all the Holy Masses of the earth for the expiation of all violations of the holy religious vows and rules, for the satisfaction of my sins and the sins of the world, for the sick and dying, for saintly priests and laity, for the intentions of the Holy Father for the restoration of the Christian family, for fortitude in faith, for our fatherland and the unity of all peoples in Christ and His Church, and for the Diaspora.

Hail Mary..."

7. The opening of the Holy Side:

"Our Father...

Eternal Father, please accept, for the needs of Your Holy Church and for the expiation of the sins of all men the Precious Blood and Water which flowed from the wound of the Divine Heart of

Jesus, and be gracious and merciful to all of us. Blood of Christ, last precious content of His Sacred Heart, wash away all my own and other people's sins! Water of the Side of Christ, wash me clean from all penalties for my sins and extinguish the flames of purgatory for me and for all poor souls. Amen.

Hail Mary..."

The Chaplet of Divine Mercy [44]

(prayed with an ordinary Rosary)

“Begin with:

The Our Father, Hail Mary, Apostles´ Creed

---

[44] Diary of Sister Faustyna Kowalska 476 du 950), cited from: Fr. Seraphim Michalenko, MIC and Vinny Flynn und Robert A. Stackpole, *The Divine Mercy Message and Devotion,* Revised Edition, MARIAN PRESS, Stockbridge MA 01263, U.S.A., 2008, pp. 65 - 67.

On the big beads (once)

Eternal Father, I offer you the Body and Blood, Soul and Divinity of Your Dearly Beloved Son, Our Lord, Jesus Christ, in atonement for our sins and those of the whole world.

On the small beads (ten times):

For the sake of His sorrowful Passion, have mercy on us and on the whole world. (The prayer on the large beads together with the prayer on the small beads is to be repeated 5 times).

At the end (thrice):

Holy God, Holy Mighty One, Holy Immortal One, have mercy on us and on the whole world. Amen.

Optional Closing Prayer (thrice):

"Eternal God, in whom mercy is endless and the treasury of compassion is inexhaustible, look kindly upon us and

increase Your mercy in us,
that in difficult moments we
might not despair nor become
despondent, but with
great confidence submit
ourselves to Your holy will,
which is Love and Mercy
itself. "

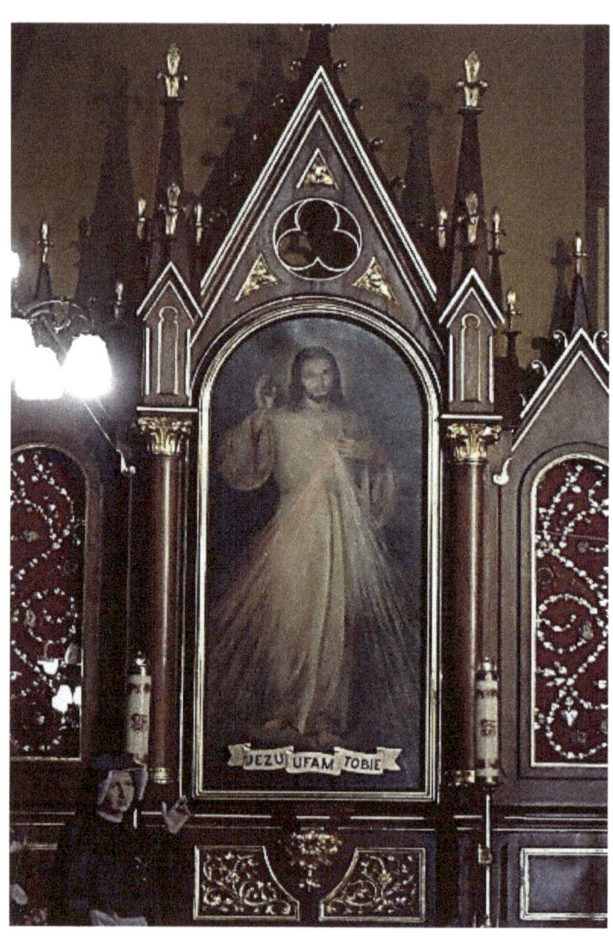

The image of The Merciful Jesus

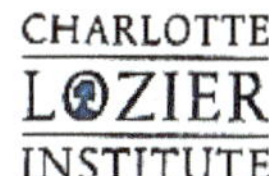

Analysis of COVID-19 Vaccine Candidates

Includes vaccine candidates that received "Operation Warp Speed" funding or have been submitted to the FDA for emergency use approval

Sponsor(s)	Status	Development/ Production of Vaccine	Lab Testing
Pfizer BIONTECH	Emergency Use FDA Application Approved	■	■◆
moderna	Emergency Use FDA Application Approved	■	■◆
AstraZeneca	Phase 3 Trials	◆	◆
Johnson & Johnson Janssen	Emergency Use FDA Application Approved	◆	◆
NOVAVAX	Phase 3 Trials	■	■◆
SANOFI gsk	Phase 3 Trials	■	■◆
inovio	Phase 2/3 Trials	■	■◆
MERCK	*Development Discontinued*	■	?

Key

- ■ Does not use abortion-derived cell line
- ◆ DOES USE abortion-derived cell line
- ■◆ SOME tests DO NOT use abortion-derived cells, SOME DO
- ? Currently undetermined

See the following link for a chart of many vaccines being tested and more detailed information about each: http://lozierinstitute.org/wp-content/uploads/2020/12/CHART-Analysis-of-COVID-19-Vaccines-02June21.pdf

Last Updated June 2, 2021

www.ingramcontent.com/pod-product-compliance
Ingram Content Group UK Ltd.
Pitfield, Milton Keynes, MK11 3LW, UK
UKHW062253290726
14090UKWH00017B/668

9 783949 222436